I0707433

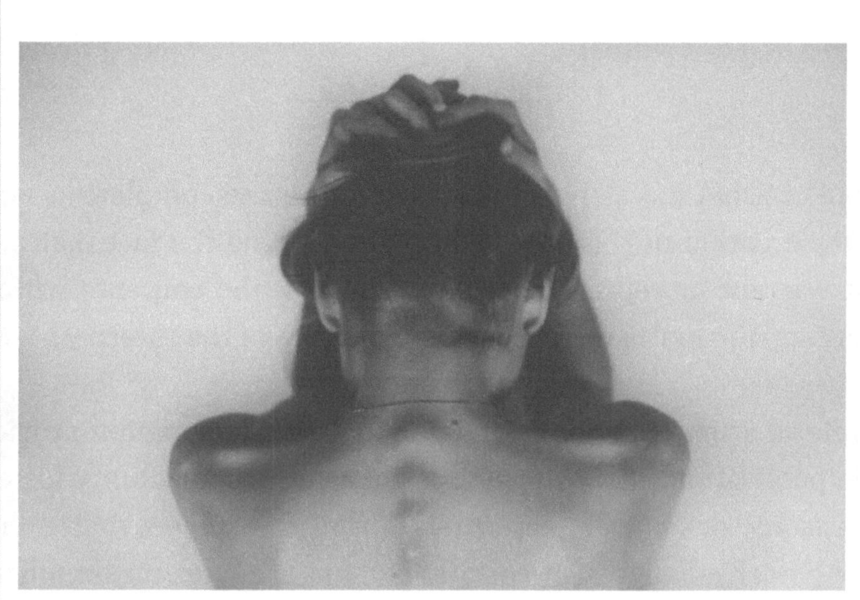

EATING UNDER CONTROL

Terms and Conditions

LEGAL NOTICE

The Publisher has strived to be as accurate and complete as possible in the creation of this report, notwithstanding the fact that he does not warrant or represent at any time that the contents within are accurate due to the rapidly changing nature of the Internet.

While all attempts have been made to verify information provided in this publication, the Publisher assumes no responsibility for errors, omissions, or contrary interpretation of the subject matter herein. Any perceived slights of specific persons, peoples, or organizations are unintentional.

In practical advice books, like anything else in life, there are no guarantees of income made. Readers are cautioned to reply on their own judgment about their individual circumstances to act accordingly.

This book is not intended for use as a source of legal, business, accounting or financial advice. All readers are advised to seek services of competent professionals in legal, business, accounting and finance fields.

You are encouraged to print this book for easy reading.

Table Of Contents

Foreword

Sound eating isn't really regarding stiff nourishment teachings, remaining unrealistically slim, or denying on yourself of the foods you love. As an option, it's regarding really feeling exceptional, having even more power, as well as maintaining your own as sound feasible; one of which could be acquired by developing some great nourishment fundamentals as well as utilizing them in a manner that benefits you.

Sound eating starts with learning how to "eat intelligently" and it's not simply just what you eat. How you eat also comes into play. Your food options may minimize your danger of ailments like heart disease, developing cancer cells, and also diabetes mellitus, in addition to fight various clinical depression.

In addition, learning the habits of intelligent eating might boost your energy, heighten your memory and stabilize your mood. You are able to expand your range of good nourishing food choices and learn how to plan ahead to ensure an intelligent diet. You will find all the information you need in the publication.

Eating Under Control
Your Binge Blasting Bazooka For Reclaiming Your Rightful Body

Chapter 1:

Introduction To Eating Under Control For A New Life

Synopsis

Here is all the motivation you would have to have to carry on with eating healthy. In this book all the inspiration to continue with consuming healthy and balanced meals.

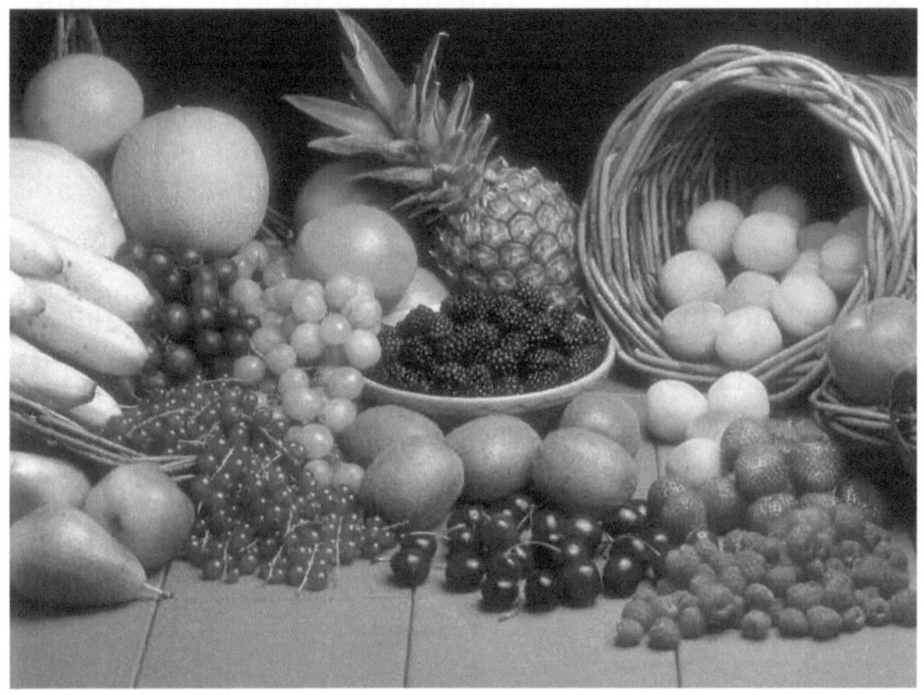

The Advantages

Let's get started with the first topic to eating under control.

Your goal is to become fitter

We can have an entire collection of publications regarding the health and wellness advantages of consuming the right kind of food. Still it would not fairly cover exactly what advantages truly exist. One of the most substantial advantage is that you gain control over your weight.

By consuming right, you ensure that your metabolic process is operating in the most efficient way. More importantly your body immune system, your digestion system and maintain functioning the way nature intended. You are furthermore shielded from various persistent illness like heart diseases, certain types of cancer, arterial sclerosis, hypertension and diabetic issues.

Note:

You should make sure you schedule a physical exam every year. Your doctor will check your weight, heartbeat, and blood pressure, as well as take a urine and blood sample. This appointment can reveal a lot about your health. It's important to follow up with your doctor and listen to any recommendations to improve your health.

A lot more cost-efficient

Eating healthy could be a path to you spend much less. Your costs at the grocery stores decrease substantially as well as you could see your bank account start growing if that's also a current goal of yours. Along with that, you save a ton of money on all the healthcare expenses you'd need if any issue surfaces because of your food binging habits.

Much less toxins within your body

Note that in the food industry, "artificial" is used instead of "synthetic". Misconception Synthetic chemicals are more toxic than natural chemicals. The most toxic natural chemical, botulinum toxin is over a million times more toxic than all of the synthetic chemicals, except dioxin.

The inclusion of synthetic chemicals in foods is on the increase. The substances may be added to food intentionally, or may contaminate food accidentally. The production of artificial foods from chemical compounds did not become a reality until the 1950s. Advancements in molecular biology, physical chemistry, physics, biochemistry and colloid chemistry, made production of synthetic food from chemicals possible

Once you start to eat right, you are much less likely to get these toxins into your body. One of the basic foundations of eating right is that you do your best to NOT eat anything that's man-made.

In addition to that, if you eat less, because you feel more satisfied with your new diet eating under control. Something else research has revealed. You will be much more aware and maybe cut back on smoking and alcohol consumption.

More active and energetic lifestyle

The results of you eating better will defiantly help you work in a much better way and more focused. You can physically exercise more, enjoy travel more, and gives you energy to play more. Here is the bottom line your life is so much more productive.

Do you think that beats being overweight and lounging around on the couch? Are you looking for the energy to be more involved with your friends and family, or simply put enriches your life.

Note:

The best energizing foods are those that are rich in complex carbohydrates, protein, antioxidants, fiber, vitamins, minerals, and other health-promoting substances. Put these foods together along with small amounts of healthy fats for a balanced diet that is sure to provide you energy all day long.

The secret to a great social life

Let's forget about fat fetishes, people who are overweight just don't look attractive. Fact is there's a strong social taboo about weight on the wrong places of the body. So, if you are currently trying to find a partner, that special person, your love handles might virtually be getting in the way. On the other hand, if you have a J lo butt, you might be attracting the wrong type of people.

I know it's NOT that simple. So, let's break it down people who can't control their eating habits and hence their weight is looked down on by society as being people who can't control their basic urges.

Believe it or not this sort of psychology does exist, though very few people will say it out loud or to your face. Once you are eating right, you will discover that these type of issues completely go away.

Chapter 2:
Basics To Breaking Binge Eating Habits

Synopsis

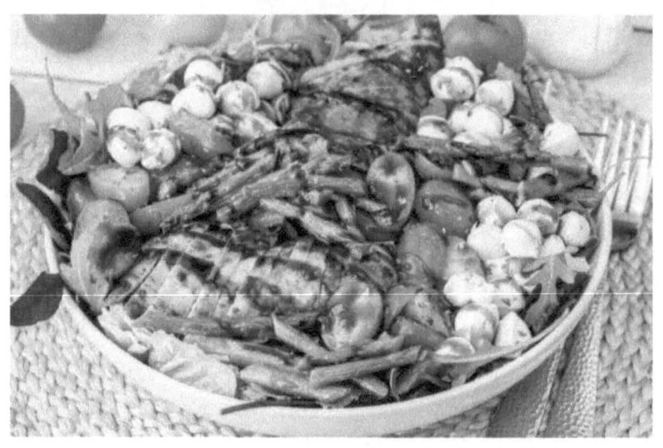

We have all been there: turning to the refrigerator when feeling sad, depressed, lonely or bored or indulging a moment of weakness. But if you suffer from binge eating disorder (BED) this can be severe, life-threatening, and treatable eating disorder characterized by recurrent episodes of eating large quantities of food (often very quickly and to the point of discomfort). Often with the feeling of a loss of control during the binge episode. Some people experiencing shame, distress or guilt afterwards. In some case not regularly using unhealthy compensatory measures (e.g., purging) to counter the binge eating. It's a fact that binge eating disorder is the most common eating disorder in the United States of America.

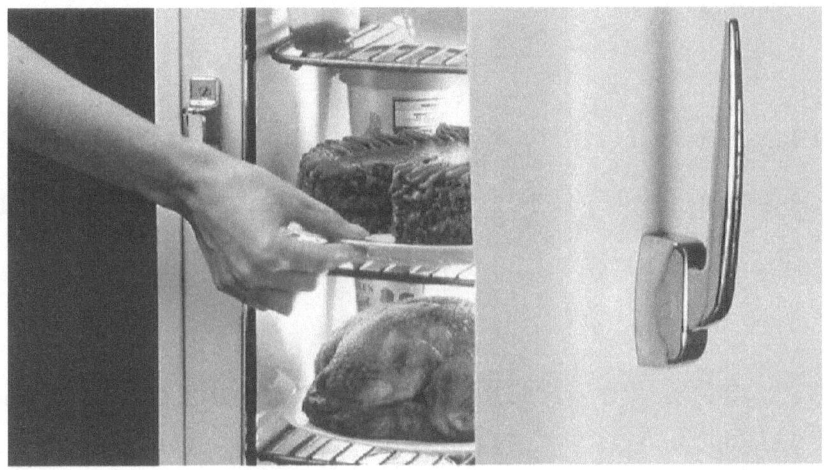

Some Basics

Rather than eating smartly to earn for it, you punish on yourself by purging, fasting, or working out to do away with the calories.

You may have found how quickly you're able to get rid of the food ingested during a "binge" by throwing up, taking diet pills or laxatives.

The vicious circle of binging and purging takes a toll on the body, and it's even harder on mental, psychological, and social wellness. You have to find some way to brake this very damaging endless cycle.

Reasons For Binge Eating Disorder

While the precise root cause of binge eating disorder is unidentified, there are a range of elements that are believed to affect the growth of this problem. These variables are:

Organic:

Biological problems, such as hormone abnormalities or hereditary anomalies, could be related to uncontrollable consuming as well as food dependency.

Emotional:

A solid relationship has actually been developed in between anxiety and also binge consuming. Body frustration, reduced self-worth, as well as problem dealing with sensations could additionally add to binge eating disorder.

Social and also cultural:

Traumatic scenarios, such as a background of sexual assault, could raise the threat of binge consuming. Public opinion to be slim, which are generally affected with media, could activate psychological consuming. Individuals based on essential remarks regarding their bodies or weight might be specifically at risk to binge eating disorder.

Indicators & Symptoms of Binge Eating Disorder

As people dealing with binge eating disorder experience humiliation or embarrassment concerning their consuming routines, signs could usually be concealed.

The following are some behavior as well as psychological symptoms and signs of binge eating disorder:

- Continuously eating after you are full
- Lack of ability to quit eating or what you eat
- Secretly stocking food to eat later time when no one is looking
- Eating typically when others are around however over eating when separated
- Experiencing sensations of stress and anxiety or anxiousness that could just be eased by eating
- Sensations of pins and needles or absence of feeling while bingeing
- Never ever experiencing satiation: the state of being pleased, regardless of the quantity of food consumed

The repercussions of binge eating disorder include several physical, social, and also psychological problems.

Some of these complications are:

- Cardiovascular disease
- Type 2 Diabetes
- Insomnia or sleep apnea
- Hypertension
- Gallbladder disease
- Muscle and/or joint pain
- Gastrointestinal difficulties
- Depression and/or anxiety

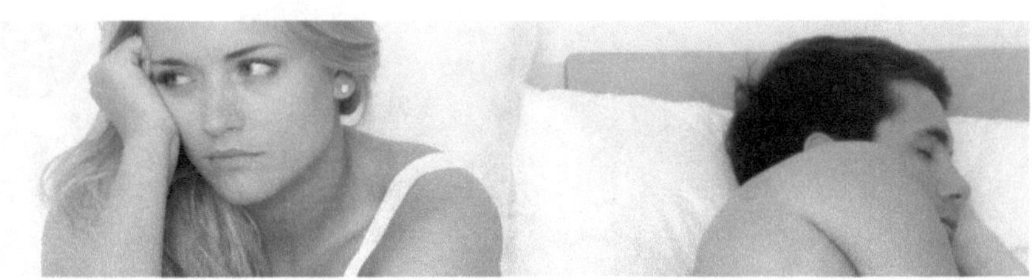

Chapter 3:

Synopsis

Cravings can be the primary reason for derailing your good intentions of sticking with a smart healthy diet program. Here are 10 simple changes you can make to your daily habits to get eating under control regardless of your sinful cravings.

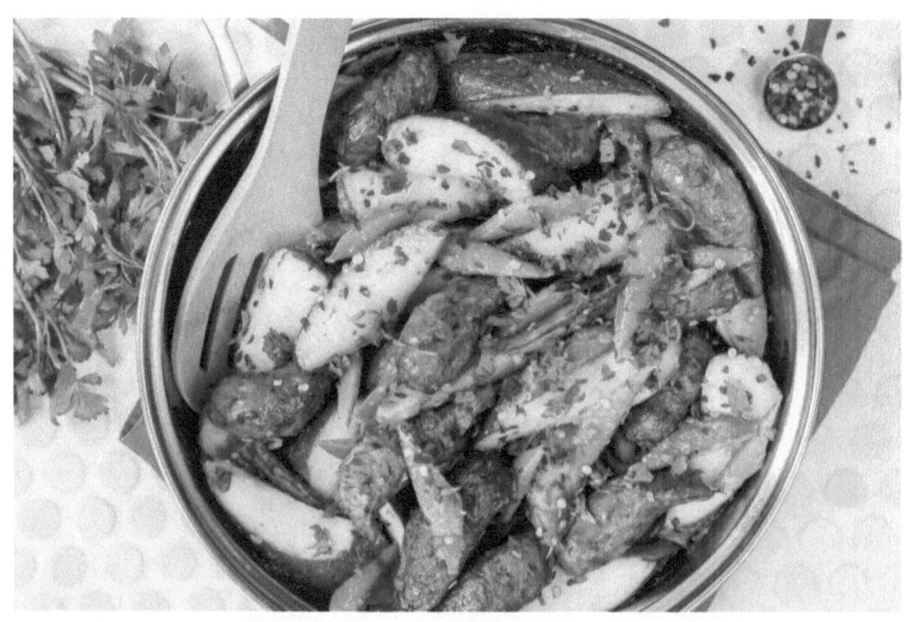

Eating Under Control Regardless Of Sinful Cravings

Avoid those tricky triggers

To control your cravings, you have to control the triggers that will derail your efforts. This starts by truly knowing the people, places, and things that fuel your own cravings and be sure to plan ahead for your vulnerable times. For example, take a snack when you go to places like the movies so you are not hopelessly tempted by the buttery smell popcorn and sweet taste licorice.

Balance your blood sugar

It's a fact that low blood sugar levels are associated with lower overall brain activity, including lower activity in the Pre-frontal Cortex (PFC), the brain's brake. **Translation** - Low brain activity here means more cravings and more bad decisions. Low blood sugar levels can make you feel hungry, irritable, or anxious—all of which make you more likely to make poor choices. Here are tips to keep your blood sugar levels even throughout the day so you can reduce cravings and boost your self-control. **Translation** – Eating under control.

- You should consider taking the supplements alpha-lipoic acid and chromium. They both have very good scientific evidence that they help balance blood sugar levels and can help with cravings.

- One very simple thing to do is eating a nutritious breakfast every day. **Translation** – Eating a nutrient-rich breakfast helps get your blood sugar off to a good start and can help keep it balanced for hours so you don't get hungry before lunchtime. Some studies show that people who maintain weight loss eat a healthy breakfast every day.

- You should integrate smaller meals throughout the day. Big meals send your blood sugar skyrocketing only to plummet later on. **Translation** – Eating smaller meals helps eliminate the blood sugar rollercoaster ride that can impact your emotions and increase your cravings.

Do your very best to eliminate sugar, artificial sweeteners and refined carbs

This is a difficult one, but if you really want to decrease your cravings, you have to get rid of the artificial sweeteners in your diet. Things like candy, potatoes, white bread, pretzels, sodas, sweetened alcohol, and fruit juice causes your blood sugar to spike and then drop, so you feel great for a short while and then you feel stupid and hungry. **Translation** – You should be very careful with high-fat, high-sugar, high-calorie foods because they work just like morphine or heroin in the centers of the brain and can be extremely addictive.

Eat slow carb, not low carb that everyone is clamming

The fact is carbohydrates are very important for good health. Here is the misunderstanding bad carbohydrates such as simple sugars and refined products are the ones to avoid. **Translation** – If you choose high fiber carbs like vegetables, fruits, beans, and whole grains! They will keep you much fuller much longer and help you with the goal of weight loss.

Yes! You Must Drink More Water

A little known fact is dehydration can contribute to increased hunger. When your body sends signals that it is hungry it can actually be an attempt to get more water. Sometimes hunger is disguised as dehydration. **Translation** – If you drink a glass of water before your meals to make you will feel fuller and can moderate your food intake.

Use The Prioritize Protein Trick

Here is a trick to make you feel satisfied longer. Make sure protein is an important part of your diet. **Translation** – Protein fills you up and regulates your blood sugar while making your body release appetite suppressing hormones.

Stress Free Is A Must - Manage Your Stress

News Flash... Chronic stress has been associated with increased appetite, obesity, sugar and fat cravings, addiction, anxiety, heart disease, cancer, and depression. **Translation** – To decrease your cravings, get on a daily stress-management program including deep-breathing exercises, prayer, and other relaxation methods.

You Should Be Following The 90/10 Rule

If you dislike everything in this book this is what you will love and a big secret to your success. Practice making great food choices 90% of the time. **Translation** – 10% of your food choices should be fun. Cut yourself a little slack and allow yourself a margin to enjoy some of your favorite foods on occasion.

You Have To Keep Moving

More research facts. Researchers has found that physical activity can cut cravings whether you crave sugary snacks or things like cigarettes, alcohol, or drugs. Instead of immediately giving in to your cravings or focusing on how much you want something, get moving if at all possible. **Translation** — Make it a high priority and stay committed to exercising 3 to 5 times a week for at least 20 to 30 minutes.

Get 7 to 8 Hours Of Sleep At Least 4 to 5 Days Per Week

Have you ever noticed that after a night with almost no sleep, you wake up ravenously hungry and want to eat anything and everything in sight? Yes? Why? That is because lack of sleep can increase cravings. **Translation** — It's time to explore ways to develop healthy sleep habits and put unnecessary hunger to rest.

Chapter 4:
Benefits of Meditation

Synopsis

Some of the time people are so anxious to attempt something brand-new or the latest trend and failing to realize that for any type of process to be successful, it have to be understood and then applied over a period of time. Fact is nothing works overnight.

The rule of thumb is for any transformation to be significantly notices is about 6 week. Some of the benefits will be notices before that as in energy and other noticeable results.

In the interest of everything, some may also ignore easy means to having a far better lifestyle, being better, healthier or simply for recovery. Reflection is among these simple methods.

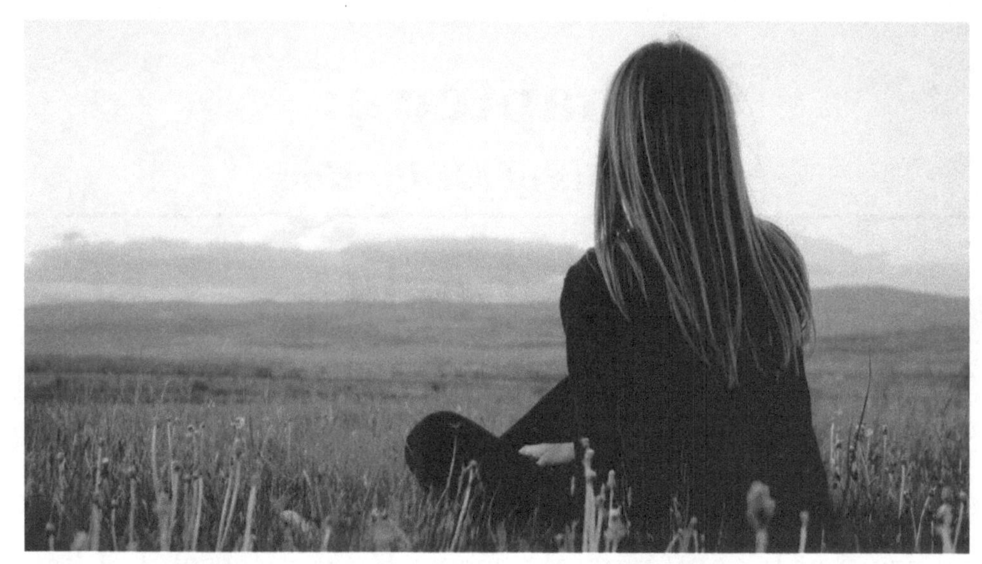

Meditate

Meditation does not need be a complicated procedure, nor need it be a religious process. Although it can be for some people helping them to find spiritual fulfillment. Naturally for meditation to work, it application and practice have to be right.

With the stressful speed and also needs of contemporary life, many individuals really feel stressed out and also over-worked. It commonly seems like there is simply inadequate time in the day to obtain every little thing done. Our stress and anxiety and also exhaustion make us miserable, restless as well as irritated. It could also impact our health and wellness. We are commonly so active we really feel there is no time at all to quit as well as practice meditation! Yet reflection really provides you even more time by making your mind calmer and also much more concentrated. A basic 10 or fifteen min breathing reflection as discussed listed below could assist you to conquer your anxiety as well as locate some internal tranquility as well as equilibrium.

Reflection could additionally assist us to recognize our very own mind. We could discover the best ways to change our mind from adverse to favorable, from disrupted to calm, and from miserable to satisfied. Conquering unfavorable minds as well as growing useful ideas is the function of the changing reflections located in the Buddhist custom. This is an extensive spiritual technique you could delight in throughout the day, not simply while sitting in reflection.

On this site you could find out the essentials of Buddhist reflection. A couple of publications are discussed that will certainly aid you to strengthen your understanding if you desire to check out additionally. Any person could take advantage of the reflections offered below, Buddhist or otherwise. We really hope that you discover this web site helpful which you discover how to delight in the internal tranquility that originates from reflection.

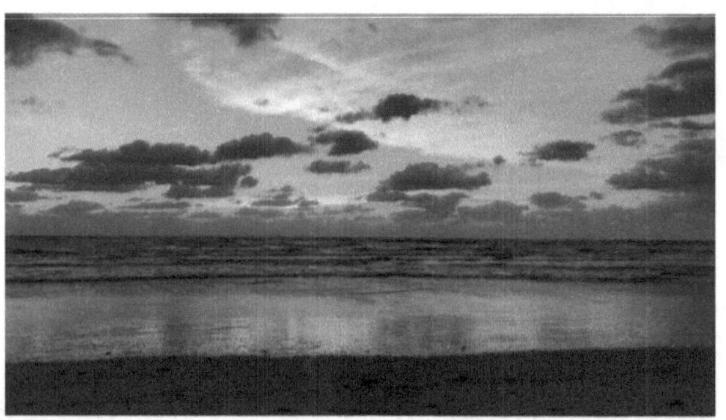

Chapter 5:
Affirmations for Abstinence

Synopsis

It's nearly impossible to have optimum living without the right type of mentality and tools. It doesn't matter what type of health you have now.

There's a particular way of thinking that you must have, and this type of thinking is what will give you the discipline to take action. Taking action is the most essential part of optimum living, and positive thoughts are called for to take major action.

If you're not ready with the right type of mentality then I fear you're destined to less than optimum living. Without the right type of mentality your health might fail. If you're considering how to achieve optimum living... you truly need this mentality and tools.

Affirmations Can Help

Affirmations are self-talk statements & better presented to the subconscious. These new images are viewed as "credible" by the subconscious & are placed in the area of subconscious having to do with the might to enhance the ability to pull up particular powerful memories with less work.

Through this particular imagery a person may develop the inner tools for the correct mentality for optimum living, letting the memories and images be transported to the present moment where they're used for enhancing mindset which is crucial for health and wellness.
Frequently individuals believe these good and beneficial self-talk memories are a fallacy and don't exist, but the subconscious recognizes where they're located and will pull them ahead for increased health and wellness.

These forms of affirmations make new neural tracts in the mind, enhancing the power to "see" these fresh powerful images. Stale images related to negativeness, weaknesses, deficiency of initiative, frail goal images and the ability to acquire health and wellness plan are diminished. When the mind discovers new affirmations the subconscious mind sees them as "tangible."

You've likely observed a basic element in those who have achieved optimum living in business and in life. These winners and successful individuals tend to be enthusiastic and zealous, in all aspects of their lives. This exuberance may be infectious, and it tends to rub off on all those individuals around them. A positive mental attitude and the might to turn that mental attitude into results are essential to optimum living, both in business and life.

You see, a positive mental attitude is a valuable asset, regardless what your goals. You truly ought to assume the habit of doing regular favorable affirmations. Making positive affirmations a part of your daily function is a great way to alter your thoughts and help yourself acquire health and wellness.

It's never too early or too late to begin this cycle of favorable affirmations, and even those simply beginning down this path may benefit from a positive mental attitude. Even if your health seems poor and you're not yet living optimally, it's crucial to display a positive mental attitude, and not let negativity sneak in to steal your thunder.

Remember that some of the most successful individuals started somewhere. It truly is possible to attain optimum living, but without positive affirmations and a victorious mental attitude, this move won't be possible.

Steady positive affirmations are exceedingly crucial for those individuals who want optimum living. True health and wellness is never simple, but it's crucial to remember that those around you, from loved ones to clients to competitors, feel your mental attitude, and utilize it as a cue.

If you're perpetually complaining about the deficiency of well-being, the individuals around you will be less than energized. If, on the other hand, you're perpetually supplying positive affirmations to yourself and the individuals around you, even in the hardest of times, they'll see your exuberance, learn from it, and use it as a cue to work harder and fix their own conditions.

It truly does all come down to mental attitude; a positive mental attitude and positive affirmations may help your health and wellness in ways too many to mention here.

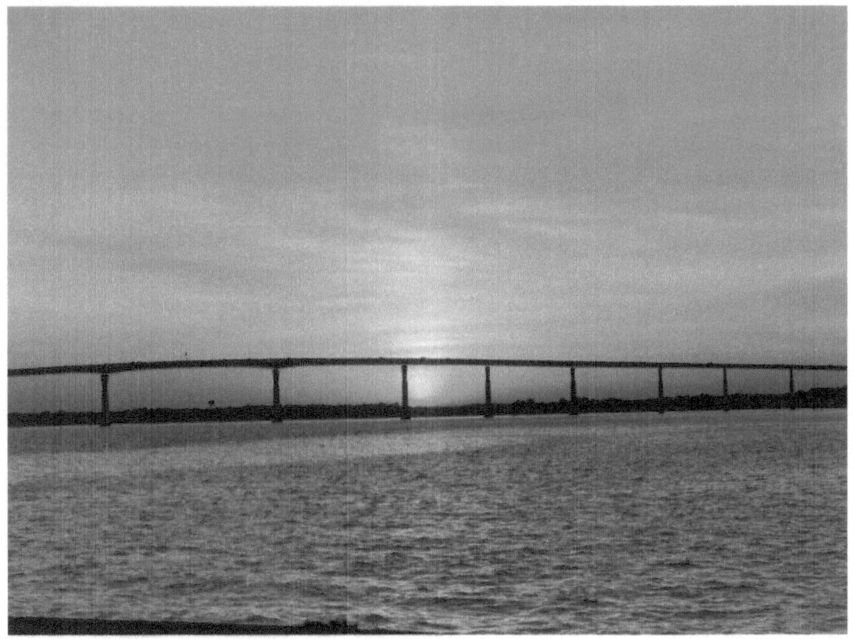

Chapter 6:

Healthy Habits For A Better Life

Synopsis

Concoct ways to be physically active. Most heavy individuals spend much time considering what they're going to eat. Ideas of what snacks, lunches and suppers they're going to enjoy and once, is what outlines their schedule for the day.

In order to bear a successful mentality for weight loss, you have to start including ideas of physical activities with thoughts of food.

Physical action works best once it's a firm part of your life, and exercise at home might be much handier than attempting to find time to get to the gymnasium.

Moreover, exercise is commonly more gratifying if it takes place in a comfortable environment, and doing it at home provides you the ability to tailor the experience to fit your individual tastes.

Get Moving

Physical activity improves quality of life

Would you like to add years to your life? Or quality life to your years?

Feeling your finest increases your passion forever!

The American Heart Association advises at the very least 150-minutes of modest task every week. A very easy method to keep in mind this is 30 mins at the very least 5 days a week, however 3 10-minute durations of task are as useful to your total health and fitness as one 30-minute session. This is achievable! Physical activity could likewise aid urge you to invest a long time outdoors.

Here are some reasons why physical activity is proven to improve both mental and physical health.

Physical activity enhances psychological health.

Normal physical activity could ease stress, anxiousness, anxiety and also temper. You could see a "really feel great experience" right away following your physical activity, and also lots of people additionally keep in mind a renovation as a whole health with time as physical activity comes to be a component of their regimen.

Physical activity improves physical wellness.

Reduced Risk Factors

Way too much resting and also various other inactive tasks could raise your threat of heart disease. One research study revealed that grownups that see greater than 4 hrs of TV a day had a 46% enhanced danger of fatality from any kind of reason and also an 80% enhanced threat of fatality from heart disease.

Ending up being much more energetic could aid decrease your high blood pressure as well as enhance your degrees of excellent cholesterol.

Physical activity extends your ideal health and wellness.

Without normal physical activity, the body gradually sheds its stamina, endurance and also capability to work well. Individuals that are literally energetic and also at a healthy and balanced weight live concerning 7 years much longer compared to those that are not energetic and also are overweight.

- Improves blood circulation, which reduces the risk of heart disease
- Keeps weight under control
- Helps in the battle to quit smoking

- Improves blood cholesterol levels
- Prevents and manages high blood pressure
- Prevents bone loss
- Boosts energy level
- Helps manage stress
- Releases tension
- Promotes enthusiasm and optimism
- Counters anxiety and depression
- Helps you fall asleep faster and sleep more soundly
- Improves self-image
- Increases muscle strength, increasing the ability to do other physical activities
- Provides a way to share an activity with family and friends
- Reduces risk of developing CHD/CVD by 30-40 percent
- Reduced risk of stroke by 20 percent in moderately active people and by 27 percent in those who are highly active

- Establishes good heart-healthy habits in children and counters the conditions (obesity, high blood pressure, poor cholesterol levels, poor lifestyle habits, etc.) that lead to heart attack and stroke later in life
- Helps delay or prevent chronic illnesses and diseases associated with aging and maintains quality of life and independence longer for seniors

So why not see for yourself? Once you find creative ways to fit physical activity into your life, we think you'll agree that the effort to get moving is worth it!

Wrapping Up

What are the benefits of eating healthy?

The bottom line is weight loss reduces cancer risk, helps with diabetes management, and improves heart health and stroke prevention.

A healthful diet includes a variety of fruits and vegetables of many colors, whole grains and starches, good fats, and lean proteins.

Eating healthfully also means avoiding foods with high amounts of added salt and sugar.

Weight loss

Losing weight can help to reduce the risk of chronic conditions. If a person is overweight or obese, they have a higher risk of developing several conditions, including:

- heart disease

- non-insulin dependent diabetes mellitus

- poor bone density

- some cancers

Whole vegetables and fruits are lower in calories than most processed foods. A person looking to lose weight should reduce their calorie intake to no more than what they require each day.

Determining an individual's calorie requirements is easy using dietary guidelines published by the United States government.

Maintaining a healthful diet free from processed foods can help a person to stay within their daily limit without having to count calories.

Fiber is one element of a healthful diet that is particularly important for managing weight. Plant-based foods contain plenty of dietary fiber, which helps to regulate hunger by making people feel fuller for longer.

In 2018, researchers found that a diet rich in fiber and lean proteins resulted in weight loss without the need for counting calories.

Reduced cancer risk

An unhealthful diet can lead to obesity, which may increase a person's risk of developing cancer. Weighing within a healthful range may reduce this risk.

Also, in 2014, the American Society of Clinical Oncology reported that obesity contributed to a worse outlook for people with cancer.

However, diets rich in fruits and vegetables may help to protect against cancer.

In a separate study from 2014, researchers found that a diet rich in fruits reduced the risk of cancers of the upper gastrointestinal tract. They also found that a diet rich in vegetables, fruits, and fiber lowered the risk of colorectal cancer and that a diet rich in fiber reduced the risk of liver cancer.

Many phytochemicals found in fruits, vegetables, nuts, and legumes act as antioxidants, which protect cells from damage that can cause cancer. Some of these antioxidants include beta-carotene, lycopene, and vitamins A, C, and E.

Trials in humans have been inconclusive, but results of laboratory and animal studies have linked certain antioxidants to a reduced incidence of free radical damage associated with cancer.

Diabetes management

Eating a healthful diet can help a person with diabetes to:

- lose weight, if required
- manage blood glucose levels

- keep blood pressure and cholesterol within target ranges
- prevent or delay complications of diabetes

It is essential for people with diabetes to limit their intake of foods with added sugar and salt. It is also best to avoid fried foods high in saturated and trans fats.

Heart health and stroke prevention
According to figures published in 2017, as many as 92.1 million people in the U.S. have at least one type of cardiovascular disease. These conditions primarily involve the heart or blood vessels.

According to the Heart and Stroke Foundation of Canada, up to 80 percent of cases of premature heart disease and stroke can be prevented by making lifestyle changes, such as increasing levels of physical activity and eating healthfully.

There is some evidence that vitamin E may prevent blood clots, which can lead to heart attacks. The following foods contain high levels of vitamin E:

- almonds
- peanuts
- hazelnuts
- sunflower seeds
- green vegetables

The medical community has long recognized the link between trans fats and heart-related illnesses, such as coronary heart disease.

If a person eliminates trans fats from the diet, this will reduce their levels of low-density lipoprotein cholesterol. This type of cholesterol causes plaque to collect within the arteries, increasing the risk of heart attack and stroke.

Reducing blood pressure can also be essential for heart health, and limiting salt intake to 1,500 milligrams a day can help.

Salt is added to many processed and fast foods, and a person hoping to lower their blood pressure should avoid these.

The health of the next generation

Children learn most health-related behaviors from the adults around them, and parents who model healthful eating and exercise habits tend to pass these on.

Eating at home may also help. In 2018, researchers found that children who regularly had meals with their families ate more vegetables and fewer sugary foods than their peers who ate at home less frequently.

In addition, children who participate in gardening and cooking at home may be more likely to make healthful dietary and lifestyle choices.

Strong bones and teeth

A diet with adequate calcium and magnesium is necessary for strong bones and teeth. Keeping the bones healthy is vital in preventing osteoporosis and osteoarthritis later in life.

The following foods are rich in calcium:

- low-fat dairy products
- broccoli
- cauliflower
- cabbage
- canned fish with bones
- tofu
- legumes

Also, many cereals and plant-based milks are fortified with calcium.

Magnesium is abundant in many foods, and the best sources are leafy green vegetables, nuts, seeds, and whole grains.

Better mood

Emerging evidence suggests a close relationship between diet and mood.

In 2016, researchers found that a diet with a high glycemic load may cause increased symptoms of depression and fatigue.

A diet with a high glycemic load includes many refined carbohydrates, such as those found in soft drinks, cakes, white bread, and biscuits. Vegetables, whole fruit, and whole grains have a lower glycemic load.

While a healthful diet may improve overall mood, it is essential for people with depression to seek medical care.

Improved memory

A healthful diet may help prevent dementia and cognitive decline.

A study from 2015 identified nutrients and foods that protect against these adverse effects. They found the following to be beneficial:

- vitamin D, C, and E
- omega-3 fatty acids
- flavonoids and polyphenols
- fish

Among other diets, the Mediterranean diet incorporates many of these nutrients.

Improved gut health

The colon is full of naturally occurring bacteria, which play important roles in metabolism and digestion.

Certain strains of bacteria also produce vitamins K and B, which benefit the colon. These strains also help to fight harmful bacteria and viruses.

A diet low in fiber and high in sugar and fat alters the gut microbiome, increasing inflammation in the area.

However, a diet rich in vegetables, fruits, legumes, and whole grains provides a combination of prebiotics and probiotics that help good bacteria to thrive in the colon.

Fermented foods, such as yogurt, kimchi, sauerkraut, miso, and kefir, are rich in probiotics.

Fiber is an easily accessible prebiotic, and it is abundant in legumes, grains, fruits, and vegetables.

Fiber also promotes regular bowel movements, which can help to prevent bowel cancer and diverticulitis.

Getting a good night's sleep
A variety of factors, including sleep apnea, can disrupt sleep patterns.

Sleep apnea occurs when the airways are repeatedly blocked during sleep. Risk factors include obesity, drinking alcohol, and eating an unhealthful diet.

Reducing the consumption of alcohol and caffeine can help to ensure restful sleep, whether or not a person has sleep apnea.

Quick tips for a healthful diet

There are plenty of small, positive ways to improve the diet, including:

- swapping soft drinks for water and herbal tea
- eating no meat for at least 1 day a week
- ensuring that produce makes up about 50 percent of each meal
- swapping cow's milk for plant-based milk
- eating whole fruits instead of drinking juices, which contain less fiber and often include added sugar
- avoiding processed meats, which are high in salt and may increase the risk of colon cancer
- eating more lean protein, which can be found in eggs, tofu, fish, and nuts

A person may also benefit from taking a cooking class, and learning how to incorporate more vegetables into meals.

Consult a doctor or dietitian who can also provide tips on eating a more healthful diet.